YEMISI AREMU- OTASANYA

PERFECT BODY

PERFECT BABY

AFTER DELIVERY

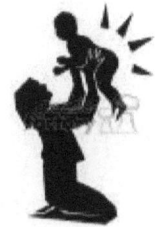

Dedication

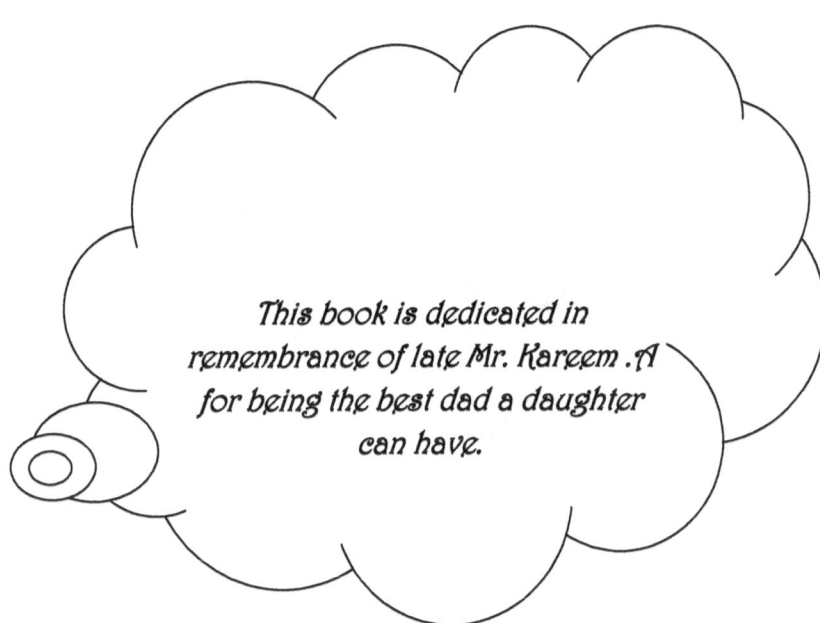

This book is dedicated in remembrance of late Mr. Kareem .A for being the best dad a daughter can have.

ACKNOWLEDGEMENT

I am thankful to God Almighty the giver of every good and perfect gift.

I also want to express my heartfelt thanks to everyone in my family for their love, most especially my husband Mr. Tolulope Otasanya for supporting me always.

Table of Contents

PART TWO: PERFECT BODY

SECTION A   Your Vagina after birth: tighten that vagina

❖ Vaginal Tear
❖ Vaginal Tightening
  ➤ Kegel Exercise
  ➤ Tightening Herbs
  ➤ Sex After Child-Birth

SECTION B   Your Tummy after birth: flatten that tummy

Understand Your Tummy Muscles

❖ Your Diet
❖ Food for Skin Elasticity
❖ Foods that Promote Skin Tightening
❖ The Right Exercise

SECTION C   Your Skin During Pregnancy and after

SECTION D   Your Hair During Pregnancy and after
SECTION E   Touch-Ups

❖ Mums Diet

FOREWORD

Motherhood is a privilege which comes with enormous responsibilities to the baby and society. So much is expected of the new mother; the baby is absolutely dependent on the mother. Meanwhile, though mother is tired and in need of a well deserved rest, she still has a home to run.

In traditional societies where the nuclear family is <u>not</u> the norm, mother has help from her peers, co-wives, sisters or her mother. The help can come in various ways; with household chores, with bathing and taking care of the baby and with taking care of the new mother's personal needs.

But in an urbanized nuclear family setting, things could be different. Help may either be few and far between or <u>not</u> forthcoming. Is it any wonder, therefore, that post partum depression sets in?

Yemisi Otasanya's book seeks to address the need for information about the mother-to-be and the aftermath of delivery. In simple prose, she takes the reader through the physical and psychological hoops of pregnancy, birth and after.

From nutrition to exercise, she pays attention to the demands imposed on the mind and body through the pregnancy, delivery and after. While "old wives tales" are not dismissed, she has prepared a handy and invaluable manual for the mother in our society. She is uniquely qualified to write this book. As a young mother herself, she has had to cope gloriously with taking care of her baby, running her household chores, maintaining a healthy relationship with her husband while juggling her diverse interest as a budding writer and social entrepreneur.

The author deserves commendation for her thoughtful initiative which calls for a wide readership.

CLEM BAIYE
PUBLISHER AT
VERITY COMMUNICATIONS LIMITED

PART ONE

PERFECT

BABY

SECTION A: IN THE WOMB

Every pregnant woman wants to have a healthy pregnancy with no complications; a healthy delivery and a beautiful, bouncing, healthy baby. It is possible to save our babies from some food deficiency related birth defects and help them have very good immune systems simply by eating the right foods, cultivating good habits and carrying ourselves in the right body postures. A mother can determine a lot about what her child will look like and how healthy the child will be right from the first day you know you are pregnant by taking conscious steps towards achieving the delivery of a baby you can be proud of.

A perfect baby is an infant that is healthy with no birth defects. Even though you the mother or your spouse has a defect that might be present in your genes, it is still very much possible to have a baby that would not show these defects. The children we bear are expected to carry our genes and look like us. Our children can look like the improved us if we live healthy life styles and help them along the way when pregnant. Once you know that you are pregnant, the first thing to do is to offer a prayer of thanks to God the creator of the baby in your womb. God has ordered us to be fruitful and multiply. "After creating the first man and woman, He looked at His creations and saw that everything he had made was very good (Genesis 1:31 NKJV)." Mark the word "Very". He did not just see that they were good; He saw that they were "very" good. God created all his creations as very good. Your unborn baby in the womb is very good. Other words for good are good quality, fine, excellent, first-class, first-rate and superior. When you are pregnant, thank God for your very good baby and then do the right things to help your baby along during development. "Every good gift and every perfect gift is from above, and cometh down from the Father of lights (James 1:17 KJV)." After thanking God for your very good baby, then start saying out loud to yourself what you want your baby to look like. Do not forget that our babies carry our genes and would look like us or someone else in the family. We want our babies to look like the better of that person. So start imagining the physical traits you would want to see. Longer richer hair, longer legs, long eye lashes, strong bones, if female, small waist or hippy, if male, strong body and whatever you desire. Then tell that baby in your womb what you want him or her to look like. "If your faith is as small as a mustard seed, you shall move mountains (Matthew 17:20 NKJV)." What ever you believe in this life will definitely work for you. "But faith without works is dead (James 2:20 NKJV)."

It is not enough to want a perfect baby, you have to work for it by knowing you are already pregnant with a very good baby, prophesying to your baby what he or she would look like, eating the right foods and living a healthy life style.

YOUR BABY IS WHAT YOU EAT

It is a great thing of joy to have a healthy baby. Our choices in life determine a lot about what we will look like and whether we will be successful or not. Sayings like

"garbage in, garbage out"

"You are what you eat"

have been proven to be true in life. If you consume un-healthy things, you are sure to have an unhealthy baby. If you place garbage into a machine that can give life, you will reap garbage that is alive and stinking. Your womb is the machine that God has created to help give life and nurture the embryo that is formed after the fertilization of an ovum by a sperm and implantation in the uterus. Once your pregnancy result comes out positive, just know that you have just been appointed a nine months contract from heaven and is expected to be good at it. Your job description is to feed your very good embryo, carry your very good embryo and nurture it with good postures and other good things.

Let us dive into biochemistry and take a look at the composition of the cell. The cell is the basic fundamental unit of life and is composed of small molecules, organelles (nucleus, mitochondria, endoplasmic reticulum, golgi apparatus and the lysosomes) and macromolecules (lipids, proteins, carbohydrates and nucleic acids). The cell is also composed of water which makes up about 70% of its volume.

Macromolecules (proteins, nucleic acids and polysaccharides) constitute 22%, lipids about 2% sugars about 3%, inorganic ions about 1%, amino acids about 0.4% and other small molecules about 0.2%. That means the human cell contains the following in order of decreasing abundance; water, macromolecules (protein, nucleic acid and polysaccharides), sugars and then lipids. This also means that to survive, the human cell needs all of its constituents in the right amount and from the right sources.

What are proteins? Proteins are complex macromolecules made up of amino acids. Proteins from animal sources include red meat, poultry and egg to mention a few. Proteins from plant sources include beans and others. Proteins from animal sources might not be the best choice for a pregnant mum with great health plans. Some dangers include mercury in marine fish and microbes like filarial worms in meat. Also, excess consumption of red meat can increase risk of cardiac related ailments. This does not mean you should completely avoid protein from animal sources. Everyone cannot be vegetarians. You can combine meat and other proteins from animal sources but in accordance with the Recommended Daily Intake (RDI) of diet.

Another important macromolecule is the nucleic acid. Food sources high in protein content contain nucleic acids. Nucleic acids are responsible for carrying genetic information from the parents to their children. Soybeans are nature's richest source of protein that can be found in plants. Its protein content can be compared to that found in meat and it is beneficial to the skin through its antioxidant and anti-inflammatory effects. Soybeans can be prepared for consumption as cooked soybeans, flour, soy protein for preparing meatless dishes, soymilk or as tofu.

Polysaccharides are complex carbohydrates and can be found in peas, starchy vegetables and whole grain cereals. Carbohydrates are broken down into glucose in the body and are used in the cells and in the brain. Carbohydrates are the primary sources of energy to humans. Complex carbohydrates provide fibre, minerals and vitamins that are important to the health of a person.

Refined or processed carbohydrates like candy, carbonated beverages and table sugar provide energy also but lack fibres, minerals and vitamins. They can also be referred to as useless sugars.

By now, you should have guessed that it is very important that you drink a lot of water while pregnant so as to prevent dehydration to both you and the baby in your womb, and to help the body cleanse out impurities. It is very important to supply the baby in your womb with very essential nutrients that will aid in proper and healthy development during the nine months of pregnancy. If you consume excess calories and refined sugars, your baby might end up with deficiencies or become genetically tuned to be fat. This kind of fat is very hard to get rid of because the smallest increase in the amount of calorie intake can make the person fat. Some people are known to have lean protein such that no matter the amount of calories they take they would never be obese. Their body has the natural tendency of getting rid of excess fat that it does not need. All this is determined during the development of the infant in the womb most especially during the first 3 months of conception. That is why it is important to eat the right foods. You do not want a baby that will end up with enzyme deficiency or nutrient deficiency due to imbalanced diets, or underdeveloped organs due to consuming harmful foods. Pregnant women are known to have cravings for certain types of foods. If your craving will do your baby no good, it is best to avoid it.

Some of the harmful foods that a pregnant woman should totally avoid include alcoholic beverages, salt water fish (ocean or sea fish), caffeine, raw eggs, soft cheeses, pate, unpasteurized milk and chalk. Alcoholic beverages and all foods that can intoxicate should be totally avoided because they can result in developmental delays, underdeveloped organs and brain damage. No amount of alcohol is good for a pregnant woman. Just imagine the way you behave and feel when you take intoxicating foods. Imagine the effect on your baby whose system is not as fully developed as your own and tell me if it feels right to consume intoxicating foods when pregnant. Knowing only too well that you can not give these intoxicating foods to your toddlers (children between 1-3 years old), how much less your baby in the womb. The presence of mercury has been detected in our seas and oceans. The marine life is constantly round the clock exposed to this mercury which is absorbed into their body. Consuming sea or ocean fish can pose a health risk to your baby in the womb because the mercury is passed on from the fish to you and to your baby which can result in brain damage and developmental delays. Mercury is more present in some fish like shark and mackerel than others and it is best to totally avoid eating them until after weaning your baby. Foods like raw eggs contain salmonella and soft cheese, un-pasteurized milk and pate contain listeria. These are bacteria that can cause miscarriage in a pregnant woman.

Completely avoid smoking anything. From cigarettes to steroids. Smoking can cut down the oxygen supply to your baby. If you are in a smoke filled room, your oxygen supply reduces and your metabolism slows down. Your heart beats faster and this results in more stress to your body. The same thing happens to your baby. Smoking tobacco and other steroids can slow down the growth of your baby in the womb which can lead to your having an under-developed baby that would end up in an incubator with deficiencies that you would spend so much money trying to manage throughout the baby's life time. Also your baby will grow up to continually manage a disorder throughout his life time as a result of your in-ability to control your urge to smoke or stay away from people that smoke.

YOUR BABY IS WHAT YOU WEAR.

We love to look good, sexy and be admired by all when ever we step out of the house. We love complements like," you look very beautiful in that dress", "wow! What a lovely figure you have", "those heels make you look taller and elegant". Pregnant women do not really receive these kinds of complements from strangers neither are they objects of desire. Instead, pregnant women are pitied and people try to assist them either with their sits in a full moving bus, or helping to pick up their falling items. In short, people assist pregnant women not court them. Not that it is impossible to look good when pregnant. There are lots of lovely clothing and styles pregnant women wear that are both comfortable for them and the baby in their womb.

It is very important to put the baby first when shopping for maternity clothes. Some pregnant women do not want their bulging tummies to be noticed quickly most especially during the first trimester and therefore stick to their tight gowns and skirts or trousers. Yet still, some continue to wear long stilettos shoes even to their second trimester.

Tight clothing most especially around the tummy area can make you and your baby uncomfortable. Though, if you do a research on this or ask your gynaecologist, he might tell you that tight clothing do not affect the baby but it is best to be comfortable. The truth is this, once you are uncomfortable, your baby is too. The uterus expands when one is pregnant so as to create more space for your growing baby. If you wear non-maternity tight clothes like jeans or skirts, you squeeze up your uterus. Imagine being locked up in a cupboard that just fits you for 8 hours. Just imagine all the cramps you will get. Though our babies are encased in a fluid bag that protects them from and also reduces the effect of shock, once you are uncomfortable, your baby will be uncomfortable too. Squeeze an air filled balloon. Your fingers exert pressure on the squeezed area, thus reducing their circumference and forcing the air upward which makes the balloon skin where the air is forced into to expand. If you wear tight shirts, you feel faint and unable to breathe as freely. We do not want to cut oxygen supply to our babies in the womb. We want them to have enough oxygen so that they can develop properly.

YOUR BABY IS WHAT YOU SEE AND HEAR

Most of our reactions to situations around us are dependent on the type of hormone we release at that particular time. Every one has happy hormones and fear hormones. Things that prompt our reactions are mainly controlled by what we see, hear or feel. The baby in your womb can see, hear, feel and taste just as you can. It is very important to keep your baby in a happy calm state so as to achieve the best positive results during development. At about the end of the first trimester, your baby is beginning to develop his hearing abilities and around the six month, he is able to identify different sounds. Most especially your voice and that of the dad. Your baby is also easily startled by loud noise. Your baby also reacts to the presence of light. The uterus is a dark place and light reflection through the mother's abdomen can be easily detected by your baby whether his eyes are closed or open.

When you see or hear things that make you happy, you release happy hormones and your baby is happy too. When you feel fear as a result of what you saw or heard, you baby feels it as well. Research has shown that babies who experience stress in the uterus are more susceptible to chronic health problems as adults such as diabetes and high blood pressure. Studies have also shown that stress in the womb can affect the baby's temperature and behavioural developments. Most show signs of irritability, depression and may have low IQ. When pregnant women experience stress, particularly in the first trimester, the placenta increases production of corticotrophin-releasing hormone (CRH), which regulates the duration of pregnancy and fetal maturation.

Having in mind that the type of hormone you release can determine how your baby will feel and in turn affect his health, it is then very important to choose to see and hear happiness stimulating things. Pregnant women should avoid watching horror movies and films with sad endings or lots of violence. Comedies, dramas, cartoons, adventures and romance are better choices. Also, engaging in light exercises can help release happy hormones.

Avoiding stress as a working pregnant mum can be quite difficult. Have a planned escape-happy-generating consolation just in case you get stressed-out at work. You can try eating something you really like. Favourite foods tend to stimulate happiness. If you close really late from work and cannot cook for your family, it is okay to buy or eat-out with the family.

SHOW ME YOUR HOBBIES AND I WILL TELL YOU WHO YOUR BABY WILL BE

Do you smoke? Your baby's brain development will be affected and he will become addicted to it right from the womb such that after birth, lack of the same smoking conditions that were created in the womb might result in health complications. Do you like partying and going to clubs? Loud noises make babies jerk. By the time your baby jerks most of the time in the womb, after birth, your baby would tend to easily scare. Do you love listening to music? Classical music has been known to stimulate babies brain. As much as possible, avoid raps and all lyrics that contain foul words.

What are the activities you enjoy the most? Is it exercising, swimming, reading, cooking, dancing, hiking, travelling, meeting new people, learning new things, or computer games. Whatever your favourite things are, they will affect your baby one way or the other. God told the Israelites not to inter-marry as part of their law. He did not want them to mix with bad habits. The Israelites were a special people chosen by God to be examples of proper way of living for the rest of the world. They were not to intermarry with other tribes and cultures. Before Christ, the Israelites were the only official God's own people. They did not worship idols and had decent holy lives, Inter-marrying with other tribes would have resulted in the introduction of bad habits, paganism, idol worshiping and others. When you as a pregnant mother indulge in bad habits, you automatically pass it on to your child. The Israelite men were advised not to marry pagan women. Why do you think God advised against such? It would seem that it is possible to pass on bad habits to our children. If you are a chain smoker, do you think you can quit before your child grows up enough to be able to copy you? Do not forget that once your child is born and can see clearly, he begins to learn from all that is in his environment. Children also learn a lot faster than adults because their brain at that time is very porous, clean and fresh, ready to learn all. Also, old habits die hard. Better to give up those old bad habits the minute you say "I do" at the altar.

Some families do a lot of research about the background of their children's spouses before allowing them to marry. Such parents would want to know if the other family has any history of genetic diseases, are murderers, robbers, prostitutes, drunkards and more. They are trying to prevent bad traits from being passed on to their grand children. If God does not want His people to mix with pagans and parents do not want their kids to marry from families with negative behaviours, then you as an expecting mum should totally avoid or stop those negative hobbies if you want to have a healthy perfect baby.

SECTION B: AFTER BIRTH

Now you have your bundle of joy. While pregnant, you ate right, lived right, and did everything to ensure that your baby comes out healthy, bouncing, happy and beautiful. This is when the real work starts. All the morning sickness, constipation and carrying that weight for nine months was just a tip of the iceberg, the beginning of a dictionary to a foreign language. Eating healthy and living right during pregnancy does not mean that our bundle of joy will continue to be healthy and happy. Part of your new job as a mum is to continue to eat healthy and live right so that your children can continue to be healthy and happy. That means you have to give up most of what you liked doing and become a role model for your kids to copy. By role model, you have to model healthy eating, healthy habits, good manners and more. There is a controversy to all your efforts though and that controversy is your environment. This environment includes all those you interact with, all the things in your house (your house is where your baby will be most of the time from 0 days to 3 years), what your baby sees, hears, eats and does.

YOUR BABY IS WHAT HE EATS

Breast feeding is the best and ultimate source of food for babies from day 1 to 1 year old. Breast milk has all the nutrients necessary for your baby's development. If you want your baby to have knowledge, wisdom and understanding, give him breast milk up to 1 year old. Some of us might say it is inconvenient or that your breast might sag and all sorts of reasons to clear your conscience of any guilt you might feel for not wanting to breast feed your baby. Unless your have a transmittable disease or have breast cancer, there is absolutely no reason why you should not breast feed your baby. It is only for a year and all the inconvenience will end in a year. Yes, breast feeding might deprive you of more sleeping time because the breast milk will digest faster in your baby's stomach and will cause him to feed at more times than if he were eating other foods. Also, you might have to bring out your breast in public and you might not really be comfortable with this. You might also not be able to go on long dates and outings with your husband, friends and family and you will also have to keep away from eating some of your favourite things while breast feeding. You also might not be able to treat some ailments like flu or cold with those fast working drugs just because you are breast feeding. Well, it is all so worth it. At the end of one year, you end up with a healthy, perfect baby. You spend less money at the hospital for common baby ailments. You get to help your baby develop his immune system fast and you also supply your baby with all the nutrients for his development.

From day 1 to 4 months, give your baby exclusive breast feeding. Make sure you eat healthy and right. Also eat well. Eat vegetables, fruits, cereals, grains, nuts, beans, chicken, turkey, and all healthy foods you can think of. Drink yoghurt, fruit juice and loads of water. Add spices like ginger and garlic to your soups and stews. Babies will suck more when they taste the spice in the breast milk. Make sure you eat your food warm and drink lots of pepper soups. Pepper soups, hot tea and hot pap help stimulate breast milk production. If your milk does not start flowing immediately after birth, these stimulants can help. Also make sure you are not hungry at any time and do avoid alcohol because it goes directly into your breast and into the milk.

From 5 months, you can start introducing other foods like pap, pureed rice, pureed boiled fruits like carrots, apples and banana. Your baby might at first reject these new introductions. Do not force him. Try a new meal at least for about a week, if he does not like it, remove it. When you baby tastes the food he likes, he would gladly swallow and will not struggle with you when you try to spoon feed or bottle feed him with the food. Make sure the breast milk still supplies most of his meal for the day. The reason you are introducing other foods this early is to accustom his taste buds to the new foods and to prevent allergies to these foods if they are introduced after 1 year.

From 8 months, your baby can try some finger foods. Babies love finger foods because they are in control of the eating. Nothing like mummy trying to get stuff into their mouth whether they like it or not. They can put the food in their mouth at their own convenience and remove it when they want. They can lick it or suck on it if the want to. The finger food is all under their control. Make sure you are with them and observing as they eat finger foods so as to prevent chocking. You can try finger foods like boiled carrots or diced apple. Find below a table with the list of all the foods your baby can eat at each stage of development.

BABY FOOD TIME TABLE

0-4Months	4-6 Months (Purees) + Breast Milk	6-8 Months (Purees) + Breast Milk	8-12 Months Others + Breast Milk
Breast Milk	Cereals (Pap, Rice, Oat, Barley)	Cereals (Pap, Rice, Oat, Barley)	Cereals (Pap, Rice, Oat, Barley, Tuwo)
	Fruits (Avocado, Banana, Apples)	Fruits (Avocado, Banana, Apples, Banana, Peaches)	Fruits (Avocado, Banana, Apples, Banana, Peaches, Water melon, Plums, Apricots)
	Vegetables(Sweet Potatoes)	Vegetables(Sweet Potatoes, Boiled carrots, peas, red beans-remove the skin first, cook and puree)	Vegetables(Sweet Potatoes, Boiled carrots, peas, red beans-remove the skin first, cook and puree)
		Protein (Chicken, Turkey)	Protein (Chicken, Turkey, Tofu)
	Dairy (No)	Dairy(Yogurt – Whole and plain)	Dairy(Yogurt – Whole and plain)

The only reason to start a baby on baby formula from 1 day old should be because the baby's mum is not around. It could be an abandoned baby, an orphan, the mother has a transmittable disease that can pass on from the breast milk to the baby, or the mum had birth complications and cannot breast feed for some weeks while in the hospital. Also, the reason while you start the introduction of other foods early enough from 4 or 6 months is to prevent the baby from having allergies to certain foods. Introducing new foods to more matured babies form 1 year can be quite difficult and they may become allergic to the food and vomit. Also, the breast milk provides the necessary nutrient for your baby but at 6 months you need to increase their diet because their body requirement increases and they need lots of energy to boost their fast growing body.

YOUR BABY IS WHAT HE SEES

Won't life be easier for us mums if our babies could take care of themselves? Assuming after bathing, clothing and feeding your baby, he would just sleep, after which he would wake-up and play on his own. No crying, winning and wanting to be carried, played with and cooed all the time. Most of us mums have such busy schedules that we allow the television babysit for us. Some of us are bread-winners and find it hard to trust our babies with baby sitters or nannies. If you must allow your T.V babysit for you, then you must make sure your baby does not watch adult channels, or cartoon channels that show violence or use abusive words. Better still, why not get your baby a lot of playful, very colourful harmless toys that can district him and can help develop his motor skills as he is trying to grasp, hold and switch them from one hand to the other.

You can also play music for your baby. Babies love music and would just sit down quietly listening to the tunes.

Once you have your baby, its time to let all those bad habits fly out through the window never to return. No more smoking, getting drunk (mothers should totally avoid alcohol), cursing, making jest of others or gossiping. Our babies are totally dependent on us. When they grow older, they take us as their role models and may choose other role models by the time they are teenagers. They practically copy everything we do. Why do you think your baby watches you always when you are moving around the house? Your baby is studying you and will eventually copy you. You are in charge of the kids and what is happening in your home. As the mother, you have to ensure that no habits that can corrupt or be unhealthy for your little one is allowed in the house or around your baby. Let your husband understand that no smoking or drinking should be done in front of the kids or in the house. Better still let him quit smoking and drinking altogether so that can he can be around for a longer time to see his great grand kids. Also family members and visitors should be kept in check. Don't allow your child catch you having sex. Some kids have been known to have sex as little as 3 years old. Where do you think they learnt this from. Its not that they understand sex or know its purpose. They just know that mummy and daddy lie on each other naked and make some funny sounds and they practice same with their older friends who have been constantly exposed to the same. If you have an older family member babysitting for you in your absence, make sure they know what you cannot tolerate. And do keep away those pornography materials. Also, have time to take your baby out for walks so that he can change his environment and see new things which can help with brain development.

Avoid fighting at all cost and do not exhibit any act of violence like throwing or breaking things when angry. We do not want to have a baby that grows up to have anger issues. When you are angry with daddy and is itching for a fight, say "husss blabla" repeatedly 3 times and wait till your baby is asleep before bringing it all out outside of the baby's sleeping room.

Now let's talk about why it is very important to monitor what your baby is exposed to. The human brain works together with our mind. The mind act as a storage and idea factory where your baby stores all past events. Our minds have an inner storage room – the subconscious mind- that stores really old memories. I remember one time that my husband asked me the password to an account we opened since 12 months and had not used. I did not remember the password but I just uttered a word from my mouth without realising what I was saying. It was the correct password. Our babies store up the things they see and their subconscious mind might call it up when they grow older.

YOUR BABY IS WHAT HE HEARS

Knowledge is gained through what we hear and see. As babies grow, they listen to sounds around them and practice saying what they hear until they master the word and can speak it clearly. We have to be careful with the words we use around our kids. Dirty language and violent harsh words should be things of the past once we start having kids. How would you like your child to use the word "bitch" to address you when he is angry? No mother would ever like that. Even though our kids would eventually be exposed to dirty language either from their peers, in school or some other place, the home should be a place that is totally free from dirty language. Once your words are clean at home and amongst family members, your child would not like to use dirty words either. Children that grow-up to speak well become respectable and responsible adults while those that speak dirty and without control end up to be rascals, rude, lawless or criminals.

SHOW ME HOW YOU CORRECT YOUR BABY AND I WILL TELL YOU WHO HE WILL BE

Some of us do not believe in scolding our kids. Some of us even make the mistake of thinking our babies are too small to scold. Well, no infant is too small to scold. Mind you, I'm not saying that you should beat your child or shout on him. To scold or correct infants, you gently stop them from what they are doing wrong while telling them softly but firmly to stop the action. For instance, if your baby is pulling the hair of an older child, you gently remove the hair from his hands and say words like,

"No sweetheart. Don't pull your sister's hair. You are hurting her when you do that."

Also, shake your head in disagreement or wave your finger from side to side while saying the words to correct him. Another instance is if your baby likes to bite. Let him know that it is not right. The earlier you start correcting your baby, the less your baby would avoid fights when he grows older. Some of us may think it is too early to start with correcting an infant. What you should not do is shout on the infant, beat, shake or jerk him. Also, you should give your baby disapproving looks from 8 months when he does something wrong. Give him the look while shaking your head from side to side or waving your finger from side to side. Then give him a hug, kiss or whatever way you know to bring him to giggle and tell him that mummy does not like what he did. This way, you would be introducing good behavioural practice to your infant at an early age with firmness, love and kindness.

On birthdays, let your little one see the exchange of gifts and be part of it. As much as possible, create time to play with your baby. Spend at least 3 hours altogether from morning to night just playing or being with him or watching him play. We mothers spend so much time taking care of babies. We bath, feed, cloth, clean them and take them to the hospital for regular check-ups. We don't mind staying awake for hours trying to put them to sleep at night when they restless. What we don't do is to give them enough play time. Spending time to play with your kids allows you to know what they like or dislike, their temperament and enables you to bond better with them.

SECTION C: YOUR BABY AND COMMON AILMENTS

Being pregnant for nine months is not what brings a mum-to-be happiness. Having a safe delivery, a healthy bouncing baby and healthy mum is what brings complete joy. After being discharged from the hospital and you take your baby home, there are a few things you have to take into consideration. First and foremost, your baby's health, then his food and then the cleanliness of his environment.

What causes sickness in babies is most time the way we handle them and expose them to the different changing weather and the environment. Simple because your baby is breaking out in prickly heat does not mean you should over expose the child. Exposure should neither be too much or too little. It must be just enough and suite the weather so as not to encourage ailments like cold, flu or catarrh. Also, avoid dust. Inhaling dust can expose your baby to bacteria's that cause cold. It can also lead to allergic reactions and sneezing.

Breast milk has been known to boost the immune system of infants. Give your baby breast milk so as to reduce chances of sickness. Make sure you change your bra after wearing it for at most 2 days. Clean your nipples before each feed either by rinsing with water or cleaning with a dab of cotton wool soaked in spirit. This is to reduce germs on the nipples and thus prevent sickness. After eating, make sure your baby belches before lying down so as to prevent the milk from going back up. Also, make sure your air conditioner or fan is cleaned often. Dust is most times trapped in these cooling systems which can circulate dust into the air you and your baby are breathing in. Trim your baby's nails at least once in 2 weeks between 2 to 3 month and every other week from four months. Dirt's which carry germs become trapped under the nails and babies love to suck on their fingers.

It is also important not to allow people kiss your baby on the mouth. Do not allow the baby's siblings or other family members and friends kiss the baby on the mouth. You do not know who has cough or any other mouth disease. You yourself, do not kiss your baby on the mouth. A peck on the cheek or forehead is enough.

Make sure you, the baby's siblings, nanny, father, grandparents and others wash their hands after handling dirty stuff or using the toilet. Most especially make sure your toddlers wash their hands after using the toilet or playing with dirt. Toddlers like to play with babies; most especially they like to hold their hands. As much as possible, prevent the transmission of infection to your baby. Wash their feeding bottles immediately after using and sterilize in boiling water with a pinch of salt to kill off germs.

TREAT YOUR BABY'S AILMENT WITH NATURAL HERBS AND HOME REMEDIES

No mother wants her baby to be sick. The mother most times feels the sickness more than the baby. You would notice that once your baby is sick, you would be so worried that you would not be able to eat or sleep properly. Some of these common ailments can be cured right at home. Yes! It is not good to take over-the-counter medication neither should you administer nor prescribe drugs to your baby by yourself. It is simply dangerous and should not be done.

Home remedies are the best solutions for common baby ailments. It is only when symptoms persist that you should see your pediatrician or a general doctor depending on the ailment. Note that not all baby sickness should be treated at home.

Below are some home remedies for common baby ailments

1. Mild baby cough:

a. Steam your baby's room with eucalyptus oil and close the windows for about 5 minutes. Allow your baby breath-in the steam then open the windows. Steam up the room again when your baby is about to sleep at night but with the windows open. This is when the steaming takes more effect because your baby is only sleeping and breathing. Covering your baby with a towel face down into steam is not advisable. This could blister the babies face and nose and cause further discomfort. More so, try placing your face over eucalyptus oil steam with a towel over your head and see just how uncomfortable it is. This treatment is also good for cold, and catarrh.

b. Palm oil drops: Pour palm oil into a transparent bottle and allow to stand for 30 minutes. Using a spoon, scrap the light, deeper red and non-thick greasy part of the oil into a container. Give your baby 3 drops every morning before bath. The effect of this treatment on the cough will be noticed the next morning and should be completely gone in 3 days. Palm oil also contains vitamin A in its natural form and is good for your baby's sight.

2. Catarrh:

Try the eucalyptus oil room steam. It is very effective. Increase the temperature of the bathing water just slightly so as to reduce congestion in the nostrils and allow for easy breathing. Also make sure to avoid dust and do not place the baby directly by the window. Mix baby methylathum with Vaseline in equal quantities and place a very small quantity on the baby's hairline just above the forehead.

3. Colic:

Soak a glove of garlic, very little ginger and 2 tablets of cafura in 30 mls of water in a bottle with lid for 12 hours and administer 1 teaspoon to your baby every night. This treatment should start once your baby is 6 weeks old. Avoid totally the consumption of sugars, ice-cream, chocolates, alcohol, sweetened carbonized drinks and sweets. Replace sugar with honey and do not drink cold water. Babies whose mothers consume these foods have more frequent reoccurring tummy aches than those that do not. Mothers that are breast feeding only most especially should avoid these foods. These foods can also cause diarrhoea in babies.

4. Fever:

When you notice increase in your baby's temperature, the best thing to do is to see a doctor. Why? This is because, you do not know what caused the fever and you do not want to leave it un-checked too late. It could be malaria, teething discomfort or even more serious issues. Try giving your baby a bath with lukewarm water after which you should breast feed your baby. This should bring down the temperature before you go to the hospital. **MAKE SURE YOU HAVE AN ANALOGUE OR DIGITAL**

THERMOMETER AT HOME SO THAT YOU CAN CHECK YOUR BABY'S TEMPERATURE.

5. Skin Care:

The best skin product for babies is petroleum jelly. It does not cause rashes and does not give allergic reactions. Your baby's skin will be very smooth and supple. You can also use some natural oils like palm kernel oil or coconut oil. The oil of the palm kernel will help maintain your baby's completion and prevent against skin infection. To prevent nappy rash, allow your baby's nappy area be exposed between 1pm to 5pm daily. You have to reduce the duration of exposure in cold weather.

❖ Breast Feeding: Vegetable Shake

Some mother's breast milk delays from 1 – 7 days or more after birth and they cannot breastfeed their babies during this delay. Take 3 full glass cups of warm fresh milk in the morning, another 3 glass full in the afternoon and another at night. As an alternative, you can take a bowl of above-warm pap with honey in the morning, afternoon and night. Your breast milk should be gushing out the next day. The Pumpkin Leaf shake below is very good for breast feeding mothers. This shake supplies essential nutrients-such as provitamin A, iron and calcium.

Vegetable Shake

Ingredients

- 50g (= 3.5 oz) of raw pumpkin leaf or spinach

- 1 low-fat yoghurt
- 1 table spoon of honey
- ½ litre (= ½ quart) of water
- The juice of 1 lemon
- The juice of 1 orange

Preparation

1. Carefully wash and chop the pumpkin leaf
2. Add a little water to the pumpkin leaf and blend using an electric blender.
3. Add the remaining water, yoghurt, honey, and orange juice. Blend again to obtain a uniform mixture.
4. Add a few drops of lemon and drink immediately.

TREAT YOUR BABY WITH LOVE

Buying tons of gifts, throwing expensive birthdays, and paying for the most clean and expensive crèche does not mean you love your baby. Buying designer clothes and hiring the best nanny does not mean you love your baby. True love for your baby is when you are there for him. You really love your baby when you breast feed him if you have no health reasons not to. You really love your baby when you care for him, care for his well being, teach him the right values and teach him about God. Pray for your baby. Pray for his now and for his future. Tell your baby stories about God. Do not say he is too young. Babies love stories and songs. Play with your baby. There are so many baby games to choose from. You can build with plastic building blocks or throw soft balls while your baby watches excitedly. Also, talk with your baby. You do not have to make baby sound before your infant can understand you. Talk to him using normal words used in your conversations with more matured children.

PART TWO

PERFECT

BODY

CTION A: YOUR VAGINA AFTER BIRTH: TIGHTEN THAT VAGINA

Having a baby is a wonderful and memorable event for the mother. After you bring home your bundle of joy from the hospital and you have been congratulated by your family members, friends, colleagues and acquaintances, the baby has been named and all is going well, then what next? After birth, depression kicks in. You hardly sleep at night because you are awake feeding your baby. Or you are one of those whose baby cries throughout the night and sleeps in the day. That's not even all, your Vagina is still sour from natural birth and you are still soaking up pad. You feel uncomfortable and unhappy that you have tears in your Vagina.

Your Vagina is a very important part of you and must be kept clean and free from infection at all times. Infection can lead to bad odour and cancer among other things. No woman wants to have Vaginal problems and to prevent that; you must take very good care of it. Improper care of the Vagina can lead to wetness all the time such that when you sit, you stain the sitting area. This is very bad and must be prevented.

You also want your sex life to continue to be fun for both you and your partner. Your partner will not want to tell you that your Vaginal hole has expanded and sex is no longer fun. He does not want to offend you. To prevent him from noticing any expansion, you have to do all you can before 40 days is up from the day you give birth. Make sure you do not have sex until after 40 days so that your Vagina would have healed properly and your body rested from the stress it endured during labour.

Also, you would have treated your self properly and would be feeling fresh and as good as new.

Below are some of the common Vaginal problems that can occur after birth and how to treat them.

❖ **Vaginal Tear**

Mix about 200 mls of warm and steaming water in a bucket with few drops of an antiseptic (detoil, TCP) and 1 teaspoon of salt. Sit on it for 15 minutes with your Vagina facing the steam. Make sure the steam is not from hot water because this can further scald your Vaginal skin and cause more problems. Do this every morning and night after your bath for as many days until you are comfortable and your tear has healed. Depending on the extent of your tear, you should be alright in 7 to 10 days. Also make sure you change your sanitary pad once it is soaked to prevent infection. After the steam treatment, make sure you wash your Vagina with clean water at least 2 times daily for the next 40 days. This steam treatment also helps Vaginal stitches heal faster.

❖ **Vaginal tightening:**

Natural birth tends to expand the Vaginal hole and this can result in reduced pleasure during sex. Vaginal elasticity reduces with each birth but there is hope, it can be corrected. The kegel exercise is a Vaginal exercise that is mainly for Vaginal elasticity. It is a very simple exercise and can be done while sitting or standing. Kegel exercise involves squeezing and relaxing the Vaginal muscles. To squeeze your Vaginal muscles, simply try to hold your urine when you go to the toilet. Hold it for 5 second and release. Place your middle or index finger into your Vagina and ensure you feel the squeezing so that you know you are doing it right. You can do the kegel practically anywhere. While washing the dishes, sitting, at the office or while lying down. Below are the steps in a kegel exercise so as to achieve best results

➤ The Kegel Exercise

Step 1: Squeeze your Vaginal muscles and hold for 5 seconds. Release and hold again for 5 seconds. Repeat the whole exercise 30 times in the morning, afternoon and night. Do this until you can perfectly hold it for 5 seconds.

Step 2: Increase the duration of holding the Vaginal muscles to 10 seconds, then 20 seconds. Always release for 5 seconds. Do 30 repeats morning, afternoon and night for 4 months. Your Vaginal wall should be more elastic by then.

Step 3: After 4 months, do the exercise 30 times but at night just before going to sleep daily to keep your Vaginal wall elastic and tight.

> **Tightening Herbs**

There is a natural remedy used in my home country for the tightening of the Vagina. This remedy is from the sap of a tree and gives full result within 7 days. It is best not to have sex for at least 40 days after child birth to ensure complete healing. The sap is translucent and is ingested through the mouth in the morning and evening for seven days. It stops wetness and makes the Vagina very elastic such that one might have to lubricate the Vagina during sex to prevent bruising. The traditional herbal practitioners that give out this sap do not tell people the name of the tree they extract the sap from but it is so very effective. You can also try tightening gels that are sold in local or online stores.

➤ Sex After Child-Birth

After childbirth, it is very important to wait until after 40 days before having sex. The book of Leviticus Chapter 12 states that a woman will be unclean for 40 days after bearing a child until the days of her purification are complete. It is best to wait so as to obtain the best results with the treatments listed above, most especially if she has tears that have been stitched. Having sex immediately can further complicate the tears and remove the stitches. Also, infection can result. Tell your partner to wait a while. Those 40 days will give you time to heal, adjust and be emotional ready.

SECTION B: YOUR TUMMY AFTER BIRTH: FLATTEN THAT TUMMY

The part of the body that gets most disfigured post pregnancy is the tummy. The woman is left with a bulging tummy and no curves. This is one of the reasons that cause post pregnancy depression in mothers. They feel, shapeless, less attractive and can no longer fit into their once tight and sexy clothing. Do not despair; this bulging can also be corrected. Though it takes sometime but surely, it is possible to have your flat stomach back. Below are the steps to follow

YOUR DIET

What you eat plays a very important role on how you look and your health. What you eat also determines how fast you recover from sicknesses, injuries, changes to the body as a result of pregnancy and a host of other things that can affect the body. Being pregnant involves a lot of stretching and expanding of the body's protein mass most especially in areas like the tummy, laps, and breast and in some cases the feet and buttocks. The body stretches so as to prepare the pregnant mother for delivery and nursing which is a good thing. At the same time, the new mum has to eat foods that can help her easily regain her once fit stature post pregnancy. Our skin expands when pregnant. Eating foods that can help the skins elasticity is very important. You can eat these foods while pregnant or start eating them after delivery.

Foods for skin elasticity

Broccoli: Broccoli is a cabbage and it belongs to the Crucifer family. Of all the cabbages, it is the richest in protein, calcium, vitamin C and provitamin A. It helps in collagen production and improves skin's elasticity. Broccoli also contains anticarciniogenics which prevents cancer and also makes it impossible for cancer cells to multiply. Broccoli can be steamed and eaten in salad dishes. You can also eat its tender stalks raw. I

Carrot: Carrots are a good source of B group vitamins. They also contain vitamins C and E. Beta-carotene also known as provitamin A in carrots help maintain the skin and mucosa in good condition. The Vitamin A is necessary for new cell growth as well as skin and hair. It also helps against skin disorders and in the prevention of cancer.

Soybeans: Soybeans is nature's riches source of protein that can be found in plant. Its protein content can be compared to that found in meat and it is beneficial to the skin through it antioxidant and anti-inflammatory effects. The isoflavone is found in high abundance in **Soybeans:** Isoflavones are a class of plant compounds. Soy beans benefits the skin in two ways. It stimulates collagen thus increasing the skin's supporting structure, thereby increasing its elasticity and thickness.

Milk: Almond milk contains vitamin E, magnesium, tryptophan, phosphorus, copper, vitamin A, and vitamin B2. The vitamin E in almond milk has anti-aging effects. It prevents collagen and elastin depletion in the skin and helps nourish the skin while keeping it firm and giving it a tone look.

Honey has potassium, calcium, chlorine, sodium, phosphate, sulphur, iron, vitamins,

B1, B2, B3, B5, B6 and vitamin C. It is very beneficial for the skin in that it works as humectants by hydrating the skin to enhance softness and suppleness. It antioxidant nature also helps regenerate the skin.

Kiwi: If you need a fruits that acts as a natural storage for vitamin C, it is Kiwi. This sweet tasty-fibrous fruits pack more vitamin C per once than oranges and other fruits. The thick furry skin of the kiwi fruits prevents the loss of vitamin C which is common amongst other fruits when exposed to air, heat or water. Vitamin C helps keep the skin firm by maintaining the skins collagen.

Tomatoes: Natural ripe tomato helps to maintain the skin's moisture and elasticity. It contains vitamin C which maintains the skins collagen and youthful radiance.

Oil rich fish: Fish oil can be found in sardine, Titus, herring, salmon, anchovy, and forage fish. Oily fish are a good source of vitamin A and D and are rich omega 3 fatty acids. The omega 3 fatty acid acts as an anti-aging supplement by enhancing collagen production thus resulting in a wrinkle-free clearer skin.

Kelp is brown seaweed. It contains 23 minerals including folic acid, vitamin A, B12, D, chlorophyll and iodine. The vitamins and minerals in kelp help keep the skin moisturized and nourished thus keeping aging at bay. The seawater in the seaweed is similar to that of human plasma and easily provides all the nutritional benefit the skin needs. Other benefits of kelp are it prevents brittle nails and hair, obesity, constipation, dry skin, weight gain, fatigue, increased blood cholesterol levels, cold hands and feet and hair loss.

Foods that promote skin tightening

The skin wrinkles with age and looses its grasp to the body such that when one looses weight fast, that part of the skin where the weight was lost might hang out loose thus resulting in loose skin. During pregnancy, the skin around the tummy area, which is about 2 inches above the abdomen and 4 inches below the abdomen, expands to accommodate the growing baby in your womb. After delivery, the stretched skin tries to get back to its former position naturally through breast feeding. Breast feeding aids the contraction of the uterus which was expanded during pregnancy. As the uterus contracts, the skin around it also contract. This act alone is not enough to bring your tummy back to its former flat state.

So many mothers have had the problem of loose skin in their tummy area even after changing their diet, engaging in all forms of exercises and so many other things you can think about. It is not enough to just change your diet and engage in exercise. You have to understand your body and know what to do to improve your muscle mass. That means you have to engage in activities that would tighten your skin and eat foods that will help eliminate fat and build up your protein.

Some foods that can enhance muscle build up and thus skin tightening are grapes, blue berry, cashew nuts, and almond nuts, peanuts, pecans, Brazil nuts, cucumber, black olives and lemon.

Almond nuts and peanuts contain protein, fat, carbohydrate, vitamins B1, B6 and E, calcium and phosphorus. Regular consumption of almond helps to tone and tighten the muscles, give strength and helps to reduce stress, fatigue and depression.

Cashew nuts are richer in magnesium, vitamins B1 and B2 than walnuts and almond nuts and are thus superior. Cashew nuts help to tone your muscles also.

Blue Berries are very rich in anti-oxidants. Anti-oxidants help mend damaged cells. When cells are damaged due to the presence of free radicals and oxidants, they mix with the cells and make the skin to become wrinkled. Anti-oxidants create opposite reactions in these cells by repairing them and making the skin appear tighter and smoother.

Cucumbers are rich in very high levels of enzymes and help in skin tightening and water retention.

Other Activities to Help Flatten your Tummy

1. Hot-Water-Tummy Press-Down

The next step to achieving a flat tummy is to do a hot-water-tummy press. This hot-water-tummy -press is strictly for mothers who gave birth naturally through the Vagina. After being discharged from the hospital, after your morning bath, press down your tummy with a towel dipped in hot water for 5 seconds. Press down the top and sides of your tummy and also your waist from the back. Repeat these 10 times daily for 8 days. Your tummy should have gone down with only a little bulge left by the 8 day.

2. Breast Feeding

The second step is to breast your baby. Breast feeding has been known to aid in the contraction of the uterus. The longer you breast feed, the more your uterus contracts. So make the decision to breast feed for at least 8 months if you cannot do it for a year.

3. Exercise

The third step is to engage in exercise. The best exercises that aids in flattening the tummy are sit-ups, pushups and leg lifts. Do not start exercising until you are sure that you are fit enough. It is advisable to start when your baby Is 6 months old so as to give your body time to heal from the rigours and strains of childbirth on it.

a) Firstly, avoid drinking anything cold for the first 8 months after birth. Old fables tell us that new mothers who drink cold fluids will continue to have bulging tummies. They say it would prevent the fat and blood cloths in the uterine wall from melting away. Don't know how true this may be but you know what they say!!! "There is no smoke without fire". You might as well do what the fable says. While lying flat on a mat or blanket with your back to the floor, raise your upper body from your head to your waist off the mat at 90° and return back to the starting position. Do 50 repeats. This exercise works on the upper abdominal muscles.

b) Lie flat on a mat or blanket with your back, lift your leg 90 ° off the floor. Repeat 50 times. This exercise work s on the lower abdominal muscles.

c) While seated upright, try to pull in the part of your tummy that is below your abdomen such that your belly button is pulled up towards your spine. Hold for 10 seconds and release. Do as many as you can. You can also try this exercise while standing or lying down.

d) Lie flat on your back. Place your hands under your bum. Lift you're your legs one after the other is scissors motions. Do 10 repeats. Rest for 1 minute and repeat the exercise. Do a total of 3 sets while resting for 1 minute in-between each set.

e) Lie down flat on your back. Raise your knees up perpendicular to your body with both feet on the floor. Lift your hips and waist off the floor and hold for about 12 seconds. Do 10 Repeats.

f) Place a piece of strong long fabric on your back while lying flat on a mat.

Hold both ends of the fabric with both hands such that they cross in the middle of your waist. That means you should hold the left end with your right hand and the right end with your left hand. Slowly lift up your shoulder and waist of the floor while squeezing the fabric around your tummy. Do 10 repeats. Also tie the same fabric round your tummy when ever you want to sleep and remove in the morning to replace with a tummy girdle. This is to keep the loose muscle in place so as to remind it of where it is supposed to be.

Mothers breast feeding exclusively become easily hungry, most especially in the night. If you have to eat late, make sure you take fruits after your late night meal, most preferable, oranges. Also, do not sleep or lie down immediately. Wait at least an hour so that the food will digest instead of sitting in your stomach when you lie down immediately. I usually do my sit-up and other tummy exercise in the night when the kids are asleep. This helped my tummy go down faster. Please do not do your sit-ups or other exercises immediately after eating, wait at least an hour.

SECTION C: YOUR SKIN DURING PREGNANCY AND AFTER DELIVERY

The skin does change during pregnancy. Some of these changes are genetic, most are caused by our diet and life style, others are reactions or allergies to what we are exposed to and some are normal. Some of these changes are listed below

- Linea nigra: This is the dark line running from about an inch above your navel down to your pubic hair line. The dark line in the middle of your stomach. This is normal and will disappear some few weeks after delivery. Olive oil or coconut oil tend to help minimize how dark this line will appear. Apply any of these oils daily. After delivery the line will disappear faster if you rubbed with the   oils.

- Glowing skin: Pregnant women give a certain kind of radiance which makes them more attractive.

- Spots and acne: Spots and acne can appear in your skin due to hormonal increase. Higher levels of hormones in a pregnant woman increases the production of the oil that keeps the skin supple which can in turn result in blocked spores. Wash and clean regularly to reduce greasiness in skin. You can also use oil free moisturizers or mild cleansers.

- Stretch marks: 85% of pregnant women have stretch marks which appears around the thighs, stomach, and breast and under the upper arm. These stretch marks begin to fade after delivery but will still be present in the affected areas. To prevent them from appearing or minimize their thickness, rub your tummy area, breast, thighs and under the upper arm with coconut oil every morning and night. Find the details of how you can extract coconut oil in page 94.

- Chloasma: This has the appearance of brown patches of pigmentation on the cheeks, forehead and neck and is caused by the increase in the production of melanin a hormone responsible for darkening the skin also called the tanning hormone. Avoid exposure to the sun as these results in the patches appearing darker and more obvious. Also use a good sunscreen if you must be under the sun.

- Spider veins: These are tiny clusters of broken capillaries appearing sometimes on the cheek. Avoid extreme conditions of heat of cold and they should fade after few weeks of delivery.

- Rashes and itchiness: These might occur due to increase in your hormonal level when pregnant. You can react to things you never reacted to before. The best thing is to avoid the things you notice cause itchiness and rashes. Also if you itch around the Vaginal area, see your gynaecologist.
- Darkened Skin: Some pregnant women become darker due to increased melanin production. Once you test positive for your pregnancy test. Rub coconut oil on your body every morning and evening. It helps to maintain your skins complexion.

Having a lovely no-problem skin during pregnancy is very possible. Once you have made the decision that you want to be a mum, then you have to change your life style which includes your diet (check page 39 for the mums diet), exercising and the right hobbies.

As a mum-to-be, you want to eat foods that would help your skin's elasticity and tightening so that you can avoid or minimize skin related pregnancy problems like stretch marks, chloasma, spots and acne. Also, you want to exercise so as to build resistance and strength. You also want to drink lots of water at least 8 glass cups per day so as to assist your liver in its daily body cleansing process.

SECTION D: YOUR HAIR DURING PREGNANCY AND AFTER DELIVERY

Some women say their hair breaks a lot when pregnant and some say their hair grows a lot when they are pregnant. Two things determine how your hair would behave when pregnant and after delivery. They are your diet, hair treatments and exposure.

Diet and your hair: There are some foods that enhance hair growth. All foods that are good for your skin and bones are also very good for your hair. Some of these foods are beans, dark leafy vegetables, oily fishes (omega-3 fatty acid in salmon and Titus), nuts, whole grains, eggs, poultry and carrots. Eating these foods though is not enough if you treat your hair badly.

Hair Treatments and Exposure: Some pregnant women are too tired from morning sickness and other pregnancy inconvenience to have time for their hair. They would rather pack it up in a pony tail or cover it with a scarf. Hair growth and well being depends on the amount of moisture in it. Regular conditioning in necessary for the hair to maintain its lustre. You might not find it convenient going to the saloon every other week to treat and style your hair. For women with curly air like the African-Americans, Latinos and Africans, braids are a good way to keep your hairstyle on for longer periods. All you have to do is wash and condition your braid every 2 weeks to keep it clean. Use oil sprays every other daily to keep it from getting dry. Women with straight hair like the Caucasians should wash and condition every other week as part of their bath routine. You will only spend a longer time in the bathroom. Also, do not expose your hair to harsh conditions of either extreme heat or cold.

SECTION E: TOUCH-UPS

MUMS DIET

When pregnant, we have cravings for specific kinds of foods. Some say it is the baby making his own request from the belly. Whether it is the baby making his request or not, the fact is that until you satisfy that craving, you might not feel at ease with yourself. The diet below should only act as a supplement and guide to choosing healthy diet when pregnant and breast feeding. Make sure you give your baby what he wants to eat but in healthy quantities once the craving itself won't harm your baby. The table below show 4 different breakfast, lunch and dinner that you can combine the way you want. What matters is to eat healthy and not be hungry. A pregnant woman should not be hungry and a lactating mum should not feel hungry just because she doesn't want to be fat.

Breakfast	Fruit Salad + 1 Avocado Pears	Banana and nuts	Plaintain + Egg & Peas Omelette	Chicken Pepper soup +boiled Potatoes
Morning snack	Apple	Yoghurt	Apple	Yoghurt
Lunch	Rice in pepper and tomato stew + vegetable salad	Wheat + Vegetables	Boiled Yam + Garden egg in pepper and tomato sauce.	Potato porridge
Afternoon Snack	Apple	Yoghurt	Apple	Yoghurt
Dinner	Pounded Yam + Vegetables	Boiled beans porridge in tomato and pepper sauce.	Moi Moi	Pasta in Tomato and Pepper Sauce + Fruits
Night Snack	Oranges	Oranges	Oranges	Oranges

EXTRACTING OIL FROM COCONUT AT HOME

Remove the hard shell of a single coconut. Rinse clean. Grate off the dark brown back into a separate clean bowl. Then grate the remaining part of the white coconut into another separate clean bowl. Add about 3 glass cups of water into the grated white part of the coconut, 2 table spoons of salt and bring to boil. Sieve and separate the liquid from the shaft. Allow the liquid part to stand for 2 hours and separate the top whitish oily foam from the water below. Heat the whitish oily foam in a pan at the lowest heat of your burner. Stir until the water completely evaporates leaving the oil.

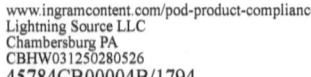